MANAGING IRRITABLE BOWEL SYNDROME (IBS)

A Comprehensive Guide to Understanding, Treating, and Living Well with Digestive Health Issues

Adams .U. Morris

TABLE OF CONTENTS

CHAPTER 1

irritable bowel syndrome

In this opening chapter, we embark on a journey to understand Irritable Bowel Syndrome (IBS). Imagine sitting down with a close friend who's been struggling with mysterious digestive issues, and you want to explain what IBS is all about. This chapter aims to do just that.

The Mysterious Nature of IBS

IBS is like a riddle wrapped in a mystery inside the gut. It's a condition that affects millions of people worldwide, but it's not a straightforward diagnosis. It's a bit like trying to solve a puzzle with missing pieces, and these missing pieces are the exact causes and triggers of IBS.

Defining IBS

First things first, what exactly is IBS? Well, it stands for Irritable Bowel Syndrome. It's a functional gastrointestinal disorder, which means it's a problem with how your digestive system functions rather than a structural issue.

Think of it like a car that runs fine most of the time but occasionally sputters and stalls for no apparent reason.

The Prevalence of IBS

You'd be surprised to know how many people are grappling with IBS. It's more common than you might think, affecting about 10-15% of the global population. That's like saying one out of every ten people you know could potentially have IBS. This isn't just about adults; even children and teenagers can be affected by it. So, it's not as rare as you might believe.

Demographics Matter

IBS doesn't discriminate - it affects people of all genders, ages, and backgrounds. It doesn't care if you're young or old, a man or a woman. However, there are some trends. It does seem to affect more women than men, and it's often diagnosed in people under the age of 50. But, and it's a big but, anyone, at any age, can have IBS.

A Historical Perspective

Now, let's take a quick peek into the past. IBS isn't a new thing. People have been experiencing symptoms similar to IBS for centuries, but it hasn't always been recognized as a distinct condition. In the past, it was often misdiagnosed or dismissed as stress-related or just "nervous stomach."

It wasn't until the late 19th and early 20th centuries that medical professionals began to give these symptoms the attention they deserved. They started to identify patterns and coined the term "irritable colon." Over time, this evolved into the modern concept of IBS.

What's the Big Deal About IBS?

You might wonder why we're dedicating a whole book to IBS. Well, the big deal is that IBS can significantly impact a person's quality of life. The symptoms can be disruptive and sometimes even debilitating. Imagine dealing with chronic abdominal pain, unpredictable bowel movements, and the anxiety of not knowing when your gut might act up. It can be mentally and emotionally exhausting.

Moreover, IBS can affect not just the person experiencing it but also their loved ones. It can interfere with work, social activities, and travel plans. So, understanding IBS is not just about medical knowledge; it's about improving lives.

The Elusive Nature of IBS

One of the perplexing aspects of IBS is that it doesn't show up neatly on medical tests. There are no X-rays or blood tests that definitively say, "This is IBS." Instead, it's often a diagnosis of exclusion. This means that doctors rule out other potential causes of similar symptoms before landing on an IBS diagnosis.

The absence of visible abnormalities in the digestive tract can be frustrating for both patients and healthcare providers. It's a condition that, in many ways, hides in plain sight, making it all the more enigmatic.

The Gut-Brain Connection

Here's where things get really intriguing. IBS isn't just about the gut; it's also about the brain. It's a classic example of the gut-brain connection. The gut and brain are in constant communication, and this communication can sometimes go haywire in people with IBS.

Stress and emotions can trigger or exacerbate IBS symptoms. In fact, some people first develop IBS symptoms during or after a period of intense stress or a traumatic event. It's like the gut and brain are engaged in a complex dialogue, and in IBS, they often misinterpret each other's signals.

The Many Faces of IBS

IBS doesn't come in a one-size-fits-all package. It's more like a spectrum of symptoms and experiences. Some people primarily deal with constipation (IBS-C), while others grapple with diarrhea (IBS-D). There's also a mixed subtype (IBS-M), where symptoms swing between constipation and diarrhea, and an unspecified subtype (IBS-U), which doesn't neatly fit into these categories.

Each of these subtypes can present its unique challenges and require tailored approaches to management. It's like IBS is wearing a disguise, and you have to figure out which mask it's wearing to address it effectively.

The Complexity of Diagnosis

Diagnosing IBS isn't as simple as taking a blood test or getting an

MRI. It's a process of exclusion. Doctors rule out other potential causes of digestive symptoms, like inflammatory bowel disease or celiac disease, before settling on IBS as a diagnosis.

This diagnostic journey can be frustrating for patients who just want answers. It often involves a battery of tests, including blood work, stool samples, and sometimes even invasive procedures like colonoscopies. But in the end, the diagnosis often hinges on the presence of specific symptoms and meeting certain criteria.

The Importance of Medical Consultation

Speaking of criteria, it's crucial not to self-diagnose IBS. If you suspect you have IBS based on your symptoms, that's a good reason to seek medical advice. A healthcare professional can help confirm the diagnosis and guide you toward appropriate treatment and management strategies.

Self-diagnosis can be inaccurate and lead to unnecessary anxiety or neglect of other potential health issues. It's always better to have a healthcare provider on your side when navigating the complexities of IBS.

The Compassion Factor

Lastly, let's talk about empathy. Living with IBS can be incredibly challenging, both physically and emotionally. If you don't have IBS yourself, it's essential to approach the topic with compassion and understanding. It's not just a "tummy ache" or a minor inconvenience for many; it's a life-altering condition.

This book isn't just about explaining IBS; it's about fostering empathy and providing practical guidance for those dealing with it directly or supporting someone who is. It's about shedding light on a condition that has been in the shadows for far too long.

So, that's our journey through Chapter 1. We've dipped our toes into the intriguing world of IBS, explored its enigmatic nature, and emphasized the importance of understanding and compassion. In the chapters that follow, we'll dive deeper into the science, causes, symptoms, and most importantly, how to manage and live well with IBS.

CHAPTER 2

Understanding the Digestive System

In this chapter, we're going to take a fascinating journey through the intricate world of the digestive system. Think of this as a tour inside your body, where we'll explore how food becomes energy and why the digestive system is so crucial in the context of Irritable Bowel Syndrome (IBS).

The Marvelous Digestive System

Let's start with the basics. Your digestive system is like a finely tuned machine. It's a complex network of organs, tissues, and cells working together to break down the food you eat into nutrients that your body can use for energy, growth, and repair.

The Digestive Process Begins in Your Mouth

The journey of digestion begins even before you swallow your food. When you take that first bite, your teeth and saliva jump into action. Teeth grind and tear your food into smaller pieces, and saliva starts to break down carbohydrates through an enzyme called amylase. It's an impressive teamwork happening right in your mouth.

The Esophagus: A Conveyor Belt for Food

Once your food is properly chewed and mixed with saliva, it's time to slide it down the esophagus. Think of the esophagus as a conveyor belt that moves your food toward your stomach through muscular contractions. This process is so efficient that it often works even if you're hanging upside down!

Stomach: The Acid Factory

The stomach is where the real digestive magic happens. It's a muscular organ that churns and mixes your food with digestive juices. But what's fascinating is that your stomach isn't just a chamber; it's also an acid factory. It produces stomach acid, primarily hydrochloric acid, which helps break down proteins and kills harmful bacteria that might be lurking in your food.

The Role of the Small Intestine

After the stomach, the partially digested food moves into the small intestine. Here's where most of the nutrient absorption occurs. The lining of the small intestine is covered in tiny finger-like projections called villi, and these are covered in even tinier hair-like structures called microvilli. This incredible surface area is all about increasing the space for nutrient absorption.

Enzymes and other digestive juices from the pancreas and liver continue to work on breaking down food into its simplest forms - things like amino acids (the building blocks of proteins), simple sugars, and fatty acids. These nutrients then pass through the intestinal walls and into your bloodstream to be transported to various parts of your body.

The Colon: Home Stretch of Digestion

Next up is the colon, or large intestine. By this point, most of the nutrients from your food have been absorbed, and what's left is mostly water and waste products. The colon's primary job is to absorb water and electrolytes from this leftover mixture, turning it into a more solid form - what we commonly refer to as stool.

The Gut Microbiome: Your Microbial Friends

Now, here's where things get really interesting. Your gut isn't just a mechanical system; it's a thriving ecosystem. Trillions of tiny microbes, including bacteria, viruses, and fungi, call your gut home. This collection of microorganisms is known as the gut microbiome.

These microbial residents play a significant role in your digestive health. They help break down certain complex carbohydrates and fibers that your body can't digest on its own. They also contribute to the production of certain vitamins and influence your immune system.

Gut-Brain Connection: Feelings in Your Gut

Here's a mind-blowing fact: your gut and brain are in constant communication. This two-way street is often referred to as the gut-brain axis. Your gut doesn't just digest food; it also "talks" to your brain through a network of nerves, hormones, and biochemicals.

This communication isn't one-sided either. Your brain can send signals to your gut, affecting its function. This is why emotions like stress and anxiety can sometimes trigger digestive symptoms. It's like your gut and brain are in a constant conversation, and when they don't agree, that's when issues like IBS can arise.

How IBS Fits into the Picture

Now that we've explored the digestive system, let's talk about how IBS fits into this intricate landscape. IBS, as we mentioned earlier, is a functional gastrointestinal disorder. This means that while the digestive system physically appears normal, it doesn't always function correctly.

In IBS, the communication between the gut and brain can become disrupted. This miscommunication can lead to symptoms like abdominal pain, bloating, and changes in bowel habits, which are characteristic of IBS.

Triggers in the Digestive System

The digestive system is a potential hotspot for IBS triggers. For example, the muscles in the digestive tract might contract too forcefully or too weakly, leading to constipation or diarrhea, respectively. Sensitivity to certain foods or the accumulation of gas in the digestive system can also contribute to symptoms.

The gut microbiome, our microbial friends, can play a role too. An imbalance in the microbiome, known as dysbiosis, has been linked to IBS. This imbalance can disrupt digestion and cause inflammation, potentially worsening symptoms.

Connecting the Dots

Understanding the digestive system is like having a map for exploring IBS. It helps us make sense of why certain symptoms occur and how various factors, from food to stress, can influence the condition.

Imagine your digestive system as a highway, and IBS as a series of detours and traffic jams. Sometimes, the digestive process hits roadblocks, and that's when IBS symptoms flare up. By understanding this intricate system, we can better navigate these challenges and learn how to manage IBS effectively.

In the chapters that follow, we'll delve deeper into the causes and triggers of IBS, as well as how to diagnose and manage this condition. So, fasten your seatbelts; our journey through the world of IBS is just beginning.

CHAPTER 3

Causes and Triggers of IBS

Welcome to Chapter 3, where we're going to uncover the mysteries behind what causes and triggers Irritable Bowel Syndrome (IBS). Think of this chapter as a detective story where we search for clues to understand why some people develop IBS while others don't.

The Complex Puzzle of IBS

IBS is like a complex puzzle, and its pieces are scattered across a wide range of factors. It's not a condition with a single, well-defined cause, which makes it challenging to pinpoint exactly why it occurs. However, researchers have identified several contributing factors that seem to play a role.

Genetic Factors

Let's start with genetics. It's believed that there might be a genetic component to IBS. This means that if someone in your family has IBS, you might be more likely to develop it as well. But, genetics alone don't tell the whole story.

Think of your genes as the blueprint for your body. They determine things like your eye color, height, and even some aspects of your digestive system. However, having a genetic predisposition doesn't guarantee that you'll get IBS. It just means you might be more susceptible to it.

Environmental Factors

Now, let's turn our attention to environmental factors. These are external influences that can contribute to IBS. They include things like your diet, lifestyle, and exposure to certain triggers.

Stress and Emotional Triggers

One significant environmental factor is stress. IBS and stress are like a classic "chicken or egg" scenario. Stress can trigger IBS symptoms, but living with IBS can also be incredibly stressful. This creates a feedback loop where stress worsens symptoms, and symptoms increase stress - a vicious cycle.

It's not just stress, though. Emotions like anxiety and depression can also be linked to IBS. It's as if your gut is trying to communicate with your brain through a complicated emotional language. When emotions run high, it can impact the function of your digestive system.

Food Intolerances and Allergies

Another key environmental factor is food. IBS symptoms can be triggered or worsened by certain foods. This often involves food intolerances rather than allergies. For example, some people with

IBS are sensitive to specific carbohydrates known as FODMAPs (Fermentable Oligosaccharides, Disaccharides, Monosaccharides, and Polyols).

FODMAPs are found in many foods, including wheat, dairy, and some fruits and vegetables. When they're poorly absorbed in the gut, they can ferment and produce gas, leading to symptoms like bloating and abdominal pain. Identifying and managing food triggers can be a crucial part of IBS management.

Infections and Gut Health

Sometimes, IBS can trace its origins back to an infection in the digestive tract. For example, a severe bout of gastroenteritis can lead to post-infectious IBS (PI-IBS). It's as if the infection leaves a lasting mark on the gut, altering its function and sensitivity.

Additionally, the health of your gut microbiome, those trillions of tiny microbes living in your digestive system, can also be a piece of the puzzle. An imbalance in the microbiome, called dysbiosis, is being investigated as a potential contributor to IBS. These microbes play a vital role in digestion and immune function, so when they're out of balance, it can affect your gut health.

Hormones and Gender Differences

Hormones might also have a role to play, particularly in the gender imbalance seen in IBS. Women are more likely to be diagnosed with IBS than men, and hormonal fluctuations during the menstrual cycle can influence IBS symptoms. This suggests that hormones, such as estrogen, might contribute to the condition's development and exacerbation.

The Multifactorial Nature of IBS

Now, here's where things get really complex. IBS isn't typically caused by just one factor; it's often a combination of several factors. Imagine these factors as pieces of a jigsaw puzzle that need to fit together just right to create the IBS picture.

For example, you might have a genetic predisposition to IBS, but it doesn't manifest unless you experience a severe gastrointestinal infection (like the flu), followed by a period of high stress, all while consuming a diet high in FODMAPs. It's like a perfect storm.

This multifactorial nature of IBS is what makes it so challenging to understand and treat. What triggers IBS in one person might not affect another person in the same way. This is why personalized approaches to managing IBS are crucial.

A Personalized Approach to IBS

So, what does a personalized approach mean? It means that managing IBS isn't a one-size-fits-all solution. It involves understanding your unique triggers and factors that contribute to your symptoms.

For some, it might mean dietary changes, like a low FODMAP diet. For others, it could be stress management techniques like mindfulness or yoga. Medications might be necessary for some, especially if symptoms are severe.

The Importance of Medical Evaluation

But, and it's a big but, you should never try to self-diagnose or self-treat IBS. If you suspect you have IBS or are experiencing digestive symptoms, it's essential to seek medical evaluation. This can help rule out other potential conditions that might mimic IBS.

A healthcare provider can also help you navigate the complex landscape of IBS triggers and develop a personalized management plan tailored to your needs. They might recommend tests, such as blood work, stool analysis, or imaging, to rule out other conditions.

A Holistic View of IBS

As we wrap up this chapter, it's crucial to remember that IBS isn't just about what's happening in your gut; it's a holistic condition that involves your entire body and even your mind. It's a condition where the pieces of the puzzle don't always fit neatly together, and it can be frustrating to figure out what's causing your symptoms.

But take heart, understanding the various factors at play is the first step towards managing IBS effectively. In the chapters ahead, we'll explore how to diagnose IBS, the different types of IBS, and practical strategies for living well with this condition. Our journey through the world of IBS continues, so stay with us.

CHAPTER 4

Symptoms and Diagnosis

In this chapter, we dive deep into the world of symptoms and diagnosis of Irritable Bowel Syndrome (IBS). Imagine you're on a quest to uncover the mysteries of IBS, and the clues you need lie within the symptoms people experience and the journey to a diagnosis.

The Many Faces of IBS Symptoms

First, let's talk about the symptoms. IBS is notorious for its varied and sometimes baffling symptoms. It's like a shape-shifting condition that can manifest differently from person to person.

Common IBS Symptoms

Here are some of the most common symptoms associated with IBS:

1. **Abdominal Pain:** This is often described as crampy or sharp pain that can vary in intensity and location. It's a hallmark of IBS and can be

one of the most distressing symptoms.

2. **Bloating:** Many people with IBS experience abdominal bloating, which can make you feel uncomfortably full and swollen.

3. **Changes in Bowel Habits:** IBS can cause fluctuations between constipation and diarrhea. Some people might have predominantly one or the other, while others experience a mix of both.

4. **Gas and Flatulence:** Increased gas production is common in IBS, leading to

embarrassing moments of flatulence.

5. **Urgency:** Some individuals with IBS feel a sudden and urgent need to have a bowel movement. This can be particularly inconvenient in social or work situations.

6. **Mucus in Stool:** The presence of mucus in stool is another common symptom. It can be a result of irritation in the intestines.

The Diagnostic Challenge

Now, let's talk about the diagnostic challenge. Diagnosing IBS isn't as straightforward as many other medical conditions. There's no single test or imaging study that definitively says, "You have IBS." Instead, it's a diagnosis of exclusion, which means other potential causes of similar symptoms must be ruled out first.

Ruling Out Other Conditions

IBS symptoms can overlap with various other gastrointestinal disorders, such as inflammatory bowel disease (IBD), celiac disease, and colorectal cancer. Therefore, doctors often perform a battery of tests to eliminate these possibilities. This can include blood tests, stool tests, imaging studies like colonoscopies or endoscopies, and sometimes even biopsies.

The Rome Criteria

To help standardize the diagnosis of IBS, healthcare professionals often use the Rome Criteria. These are a set of guidelines that help determine if a person's symptoms align with IBS. To meet the criteria, symptoms must have been present for a specific duration (usually at least six months) and meet specific criteria for frequency and intensity.

However, it's important to note that not everyone with IBS fits neatly into these criteria. Some individuals have symptoms that don't precisely match the Rome Criteria but still experience significant discomfort and disruption in their daily lives.

The Importance of a Thorough Evaluation

Getting a proper diagnosis is crucial for several reasons. First and foremost, it helps rule out more serious conditions that might mimic IBS. Second, it can provide much-needed validation for individuals who have been suffering from unexplained symptoms. Third, a diagnosis can guide treatment and management strategies.

Types of IBS

As if the diagnostic process wasn't complex enough, IBS is further divided into subtypes based on the predominant bowel habits. These subtypes help tailor treatment and management approaches. Here are the main subtypes:

1. **IBS with Constipation (IBS-C):** Characterized by more frequent episodes of

constipation and abdominal discomfort.

2. **IBS with Diarrhea (IBS-D):** Marked by episodes of diarrhea and urgency.

3. **Mixed IBS (IBS-M):** Involves a combination of both constipation and diarrhea.

4. **Unspecified IBS (IBS-U):** When symptoms don't fit neatly into one of the above categories.

IBS as a Chronic Condition

It's essential to recognize that IBS is a chronic condition, which means it tends to persist over time. Symptoms can come and go, and their severity can vary, but IBS rarely disappears completely.

The Gut-Brain Connection in IBS Symptoms

Remember the gut-brain connection we discussed earlier? It's essential here too. Stress and emotions can significantly impact IBS symptoms. Some individuals find that their symptoms worsen during times of high stress, anxiety, or emotional upheaval. This is why managing stress is often a key component of IBS management.

The Role of Diet in IBS Symptoms

Diet plays a pivotal role in IBS symptoms. Certain foods can trigger or exacerbate symptoms in susceptible individuals. One dietary approach that has gained attention is the low FODMAP diet. FODMAPs are types of carbohydrates that are poorly absorbed in the small intestine and can ferment in the colon, leading to gas and bloating.

However, it's crucial to approach dietary changes under the guidance of a healthcare provider or dietitian, as eliminating certain foods can have nutritional consequences. Additionally, dietary triggers can vary widely between individuals, making personalized dietary advice essential.

Treatment and Management of IBS Symptoms

Managing IBS symptoms often involves a multifaceted approach. Here are some key components:

1. **Dietary Modifications:** As mentioned, certain dietary changes, such as a low FODMAP diet, might be recommended. It's essential

to do this with the guidance of a healthcare provider or dietitian.

2. **Stress Management:** Stress reduction techniques like mindfulness, meditation, or yoga can help reduce the impact of stress on IBS symptoms.

3. **Medications:** Depending on your specific symptoms, medications may be prescribed. These can include antispasmodic drugs, laxatives, anti-diarrheal medications, or even medications that target pain and discomfort.

4. **Probiotics:** Some individuals find relief from IBS symptoms by taking probiotics, which can help promote a healthier gut microbiome.

5. **Lifestyle Changes:** Simple lifestyle adjustments, such as regular exercise and adequate sleep, can also contribute to symptom management.

6. **Psychological Therapies:** In cases where stress and emotions play a significant role, psychological therapies like cognitive-behavioral

therapy (CBT) can be beneficial.

The Impact of IBS on Quality of Life

Living with IBS can be challenging, and it can significantly impact a person's quality of life. The unpredictable nature of symptoms, the discomfort, and the need to plan activities around bathroom access can be emotionally and socially taxing.

Conclusion: Navigating the World of IBS Symptoms and Diagnosis

As we conclude this chapter, it's crucial to understand that IBS isn't just about digestive discomfort. It's a complex condition with a wide range of symptoms, and getting an accurate diagnosis is a critical step in managing it effectively.

In the chapters to come, we'll explore various aspects of IBS management, including medications, alternative therapies, and lifestyle changes. Our goal is to provide you with the knowledge and tools you need to navigate the world of IBS and improve your quality of life. So, stay with us as

we continue our journey through
the realm of Irritable Bowel
Syndrome.

CHAPTER 5

Types of IBS

Welcome to Chapter 5, where we're going to delve into the different types of Irritable Bowel Syndrome (IBS). This is like uncovering the unique personalities of IBS, each with its own set of symptoms and challenges. Let's explore the various types and what makes each one distinct.

IBS with Constipation (IBS-C)

Imagine your digestive system hitting the brakes more often than it should. That's what it feels like for individuals with IBS-C. In this subtype, constipation is the primary issue, and it can be a real, well, pain in the gut.

The Main Features of IBS-C:

1. **Infrequent Bowel Movements:** People with IBS-C often have less frequent bowel movements than they should. They might go three days or even longer between trips to the bathroom.

2. **Hard, Dry Stools:** When they do finally go, the stools are usually hard, dry, and difficult to pass. It can feel like trying to push through a brick wall.

3. **Straining:** Straining during bowel movements is common, and it can lead to discomfort and even hemorrhoids.

4. **Bloating and Discomfort:** Bloating and abdominal discomfort often accompany constipation in IBS-C.

IBS with Diarrhea (IBS-D)

Now, picture the opposite scenario. Your digestive system decides to hit the gas pedal, and you're making more trips to the bathroom than you'd like. That's the world of IBS-D, where diarrhea takes center stage.

The Main Features of IBS-D:

1. **Frequent Bowel Movements:** Individuals with IBS-D typically experience more frequent bowel movements than normal. It can be several times a day or even more.

2. **Urgency:** There's often a sense of urgency, a feeling

that you need to find a bathroom right now. It can be particularly challenging when you're away from home.

3. **Loose Stools:** Stools in IBS-D are loose and watery, which can lead to dehydration if not managed carefully.

4. **Cramping:** Abdominal cramping and discomfort are common and can be quite painful.

Mixed IBS (IBS-M)

Now, what if you're stuck in a constant tug-of-war between

constipation and diarrhea? That's the realm of Mixed IBS, or IBS-M. In this subtype, your digestive system can't seem to make up its mind, and symptoms swing between the two extremes.

The Main Features of IBS-M:

1. **Alternating Symptoms:** People with IBS-M experience alternating bouts of constipation and diarrhea. One day, it might be hard, dry stools, and the next, it's urgent trips to the bathroom.

2. **Unpredictability:** The unpredictability of symptoms can be

particularly frustrating and challenging to manage.

3. **Bloating and Cramping:** As with other subtypes, abdominal bloating and cramping are common.

Unspecified IBS (IBS-U)

Now, what if your symptoms don't neatly fit into one of these categories? That's where Unspecified IBS, or IBS-U, comes into play. In IBS-U, the symptoms might not align with the classic features of IBS-C, IBS-D, or IBS-M.

The Main Features of IBS-U:

1. **Varied Symptoms:** Symptoms in IBS-U can be varied and might not follow a specific pattern. This can make diagnosis and management a bit more challenging.

2. **Individualized Experience:** IBS-U often represents an individualized experience, with symptoms that don't neatly fit into one of the other subtypes.

Why Subtypes Matter

You might wonder why these subtypes matter. Well, understanding which subtype of

IBS you have can help guide treatment and management strategies. It's like having a roadmap that tells you where you're starting from and where you want to go.

Treatment and Management by Subtype

For IBS-C:

1. **Dietary Fiber:** Increasing dietary fiber intake can help regulate bowel movements and alleviate constipation.

2. **Hydration:** Drinking plenty of water is essential to

soften stools and make them easier to pass.

3. **Laxatives:** In some cases, laxatives may be recommended, but they should be used under medical supervision.

For IBS-D:

1. **Dietary Changes:** Avoiding trigger foods that worsen diarrhea can be helpful. Common triggers include spicy foods, caffeine, and artificial sweeteners.

2. **Antidiarrheal Medications:** Over-the-counter antidiarrheal

medications like loperamide can provide relief.

3. **Probiotics:** Some individuals find that probiotics help regulate bowel movements and reduce diarrhea.

For IBS-M:

1. **Dietary Management:** A balanced diet with a focus on fiber can help regulate bowel habits. Identifying specific triggers through a food diary can also be useful.

2. **Medications:** Depending on the predominant symptoms, medications like

antispasmodics or antidiarrheals may be recommended.

For IBS-U:

Treatment for IBS-U often involves a more individualized approach. It might require a combination of dietary changes, stress management techniques, and possibly medications based on the specific symptoms you experience.

Personalized Approach

Remember, IBS management is not one-size-fits-all. Your subtype, symptoms, and triggers are unique to you. This is why a personalized approach, often guided by a healthcare provider or dietitian, is so crucial.

Beyond Subtypes: The Impact of Stress and Lifestyle

It's also important to recognize that stress and lifestyle factors can play a significant role in all subtypes of IBS. Stress reduction techniques like mindfulness, meditation, or yoga can help alleviate symptoms.

Lifestyle factors like regular exercise, staying hydrated, and getting enough sleep can also

make a big difference in IBS
management. These practices
promote overall digestive health
and can help reduce the impact of
symptoms.

Conclusion: Navigating the World of IBS Subtypes

As we wrap up this chapter, it's
important to remember that IBS is
not a one-size-fits-all condition.
The subtypes of IBS help us
understand the diverse ways this
condition can manifest and guide
us toward more effective
treatment and management.

In the chapters ahead, we'll explore various aspects of managing IBS, including medications, psychological therapies, and dietary strategies. Our journey through the world of Irritable Bowel Syndrome continues, and we're here to provide you with the knowledge and tools you need to navigate it successfully. So, stay with us as we continue our exploration.

CHAPTER 6

Management and Coping Strategies for IBS

Welcome to Chapter 6, where we're going to dive into the practical aspects of managing and coping with Irritable Bowel Syndrome (IBS). Think of this chapter as your toolbox, filled with strategies and techniques to help you navigate the challenges of living with IBS effectively.

A Holistic Approach

Managing IBS often involves a holistic approach that addresses various aspects of your life. It's not just about treating physical symptoms; it's also about managing the emotional and lifestyle factors that can impact IBS.

Dietary Strategies

Diet plays a significant role in IBS management, and what works for one person may not work for another. Here are some dietary strategies that can be helpful:

1. **Low FODMAP Diet:** This dietary approach involves

reducing the consumption of fermentable carbohydrates known as FODMAPs. It can be highly effective, especially for those with IBS-D or IBS-M. However, it's essential to undertake this diet under the guidance of a healthcare provider or dietitian, as it can be complex to follow.

2. Food Diary: Keeping a food diary can help identify specific trigger foods that worsen your symptoms. Note what you eat and how it affects your digestion to pinpoint problem foods.

3. Fiber: Adequate fiber intake is crucial for regular bowel movements. Soluble fiber, found in foods like oats and legumes, can be gentler on the gut and may help regulate bowel habits.

4. Probiotics: Some individuals with IBS find relief by taking probiotics, which can help balance the gut microbiome. However, the effectiveness can vary from person to person, so it's essential to choose the right probiotic strain and discuss it with your healthcare provider.

Stress Management

Stress and IBS often go hand in hand, creating a vicious cycle where stress worsens symptoms, and symptoms increase stress. Managing stress can be a game-changer in IBS management. Here are some stress-reduction techniques to consider:

1.   Mindfulness and Meditation: Mindfulness practices and meditation can help you stay grounded and reduce the impact of stress on your digestive system.

2. Deep Breathing: Simple deep breathing exercises can be done anywhere and anytime you feel stressed. They help activate the relaxation response in your body.

3. Yoga: Yoga combines physical postures, breath control, and mindfulness, making it an excellent practice for reducing stress and improving overall well-being.

4. Cognitive-Behavioral Therapy (CBT): CBT is a psychological therapy that can help you identify and change thought patterns and behaviors that contribute to stress and anxiety.

Lifestyle Adjustments

Certain lifestyle changes can make a big difference in managing IBS.

Here are some key adjustments to consider:

1. Regular Exercise: Exercise promotes overall digestive health and can help regulate bowel movements. Aim for at least 30 minutes of moderate exercise most days of the week.

2. Hydration: Staying adequately hydrated is essential, especially if you experience diarrhea. Dehydration can worsen symptoms, so make sure you're drinking enough water throughout the day.

3. Sleep: Getting enough restorative sleep is crucial for overall health and can help reduce stress. Create a sleep-friendly environment and establish a regular sleep routine.

4. Bathroom Access: Plan your day to ensure easy access to a bathroom when needed. This can help reduce anxiety about finding a restroom in public places.

Medications for Symptom Relief

In some cases, medications may be necessary to manage specific symptoms of IBS. It's essential to discuss these options with your healthcare provider, as they can recommend the most suitable treatments based on your subtype and symptoms. Here are some medication options:

1. **Antispasmodic Medications:** These drugs can help relax the muscles in your digestive tract, reducing cramping and pain.

2. Antidiarrheal Medications: Over-the-counter antidiarrheal medications like loperamide can be useful for managing diarrhea.

3. Laxatives: For those with IBS-C, laxatives may be prescribed to alleviate constipation. However, these should be used under medical supervision.

4. Pain Medications: In some cases, pain medications may be prescribed to manage severe abdominal pain.

Psychological Therapies

Mental health and emotional well-being are essential components of managing IBS. Here are two psychological therapies that can be beneficial:

1.   **Cognitive-Behavioral Therapy (CBT):** CBT can help you identify and modify thought patterns and behaviors that contribute to stress and anxiety, both of which can exacerbate IBS symptoms.

2.   **Gut-Directed Hypnotherapy:** This specialized form of hypnotherapy focuses on the gut-brain connection and can help reduce pain and discomfort in people with IBS.

Support Groups

Living with IBS can be challenging, and you're not alone

in this journey. Support groups, either in person or online, can provide a sense of community and a safe space to share experiences and coping strategies. Connecting with others who understand what you're going through can be incredibly empowering.

Alternative and Complementary Therapies

Some individuals with IBS find relief through alternative and complementary therapies. While these approaches may not be a standalone solution, they can complement conventional treatments. Here are a few options to consider:

1. **Acupuncture:** Acupuncture involves the insertion of thin needles into specific points on the body and is believed to help regulate energy flow and alleviate symptoms.

2. **Herbal Remedies:** Certain herbal supplements, like peppermint oil capsules or ginger, have shown promise in reducing IBS symptoms for some individuals.

3. **Hypnotherapy:** Hypnotherapy can help reduce

pain and discomfort in people with IBS by addressing the gut-brain connection.

Patient Education and Self-Advocacy

Understanding your condition and being your advocate is a critical part of managing IBS. Educate yourself about IBS, its subtypes, and the various treatment options available. Keep a symptom diary to track patterns and triggers. And don't hesitate to communicate openly with your healthcare provider about your symptoms and concerns.

Conclusion: Empowering Yourself in IBS Management

As we conclude this chapter, remember that managing IBS is about empowerment. It's about finding the right combination of strategies and techniques that work for you. It's about recognizing that living with IBS doesn't define you; it's just one aspect of your life.

In the chapters ahead, we'll continue to explore various aspects of living with IBS, from dietary considerations to the emotional impact of the condition. Our goal is to provide you with the knowledge and tools you need to thrive, despite the challenges of IBS. So, stay with us as we continue our journey through the world of Irritable Bowel Syndrome.

CHAPTER 7

Diet and Nutrition for IBS

Welcome to Chapter 7, where we'll explore the crucial role that diet and nutrition play in managing Irritable Bowel Syndrome (IBS). Think of this chapter as your dietary compass, guiding you through the often complex landscape of IBS-friendly eating.

Understanding the Impact of Diet

Diet is a central player in the world of IBS. Certain foods can trigger or exacerbate symptoms, while others can help soothe your digestive system. Understanding your dietary triggers and adopting a balanced eating plan can significantly improve your quality of life with IBS.

Low FODMAP Diet

One dietary approach that has gained attention in IBS management is the Low FODMAP diet. FODMAPs are fermentable carbohydrates found in many foods. In some individuals with IBS, these carbohydrates are poorly absorbed in the small intestine and can lead to symptoms like bloating, gas, and diarrhea.

What Are FODMAPs?

FODMAP stands for "Fermentable Oligosaccharides, Disaccharides, Monosaccharides, and Polyols." These are types of carbohydrates that are osmotically active, meaning they draw water into the digestive tract. This can lead to increased gas production and changes in bowel habits.

Common High-FODMAP Foods:

- **Fructans:** Found in wheat, onions, garlic, and some fruits.

- **Lactose:** Present in dairy products like milk and yogurt.

- **Fructose:** Found in honey, certain fruits, and high-fructose corn syrup.

- **Polyols:** These are sugar alcohols found in some fruits, vegetables, and sugar-free gums and candies.

- **Galacto-oligosaccharides (GOS):** Found in legumes like lentils and chickpeas.

How Does the Low FODMAP Diet Work?

The Low FODMAP diet involves reducing your intake of high-FODMAP foods and then gradually reintroducing them to identify your specific triggers. It typically has three phases:

1. **Elimination Phase:** During this phase, you significantly reduce your intake of high-FODMAP foods to minimize symptoms. This phase usually lasts 2-6 weeks.

2. **Reintroduction Phase:** After the elimination phase,

you systematically reintroduce high-FODMAP foods one at a time to identify which ones trigger your symptoms.

3. **Personalization Phase:** Based on your reactions during the reintroduction phase, you create a personalized long-term eating plan that avoids your specific triggers but includes as many low-FODMAP foods as possible.

Working with a Dietitian

The Low FODMAP diet is complex and should be undertaken with the guidance of a registered dietitian or healthcare provider. They can help you create a personalized plan, ensure you meet your nutritional needs, and navigate the various phases of the diet safely.

Other Dietary Considerations for IBS

While the Low FODMAP diet has shown promise for many individuals with IBS, it's not the only dietary consideration. Here are some other dietary strategies to keep in mind:

1. **Fiber Intake:** Adequate fiber intake is crucial for regular bowel

movements. Soluble fiber, found in foods like oats, beans, and certain fruits, can be gentler on the gut and may help regulate bowel habits.

2. Avoid Trigger Foods: Identify and avoid specific trigger foods that worsen your symptoms. Common triggers include spicy foods, caffeine, alcohol, and artificial sweeteners.

3. Smaller, Frequent Meals: Instead of three large meals, consider eating smaller, more frequent meals throughout the day. This can help prevent overloading your digestive system.

4. Food Sensitivities: Some individuals with IBS might have additional food sensitivities beyond FODMAPs. Keeping a food diary can help pinpoint these sensitivities.

5. Stay Hydrated: Drinking plenty of water is essential, especially if you experience diarrhea, as it can lead to dehydration.

6. Balanced Eating: Strive for a balanced diet that includes a variety of foods from all food groups. This can help ensure you get the nutrients your body needs.

7. Probiotics: Probiotics, which contain beneficial bacteria, can help regulate the gut microbiome and reduce symptoms for some individuals with IBS. Talk to your healthcare provider about whether they might be right for you.

8. Mindful Eating: Pay attention to your eating habits. Eating too quickly or when stressed can lead to swallowing air and worsening symptoms.

9. Alcohol and Caffeine: Limit or avoid alcohol and caffeine, as they can be irritants to the digestive tract.

10. Be Patient: Dietary changes can take time to show their full effect. Give your body time to adjust to a new eating plan.

Alcohol, Caffeine, and IBS

Alcohol and caffeine can be problematic for individuals with IBS. Alcohol can irritate the gastrointestinal tract, leading to symptoms like diarrhea and abdominal pain. Caffeine, found in coffee, tea, and some soft drinks, can stimulate the gut and lead to urgency and diarrhea in some people.

Managing Social Situations

Eating out or attending social gatherings can be challenging when you have IBS. Here are some tips for managing these situations:

1. Plan Ahead: Look at menus in advance and choose restaurants that offer options aligned with your dietary needs.

2. Communicate: Don't hesitate to communicate your dietary restrictions or preferences to the restaurant staff. Many restaurants are accommodating and can make adjustments to their dishes.

3. Bring Snacks: If you're unsure about food options,

consider bringing a small snack or meal with you.

4. Be Mindful: Pay attention to portion sizes and avoid overeating, which can trigger symptoms.

Emotional Impact of Diet and Nutrition in IBS

Managing IBS can be emotionally challenging, especially when dietary restrictions affect your social life or cause frustration. It's essential to recognize the emotional impact of diet and nutrition and seek support when needed. Here are a few key points:

1. **Emotional Eating:** Be mindful of emotional eating patterns. Stress or frustration can lead to unhealthy food choices, which can exacerbate symptoms.

2. **Seek Support:** If you're struggling with the emotional aspects of dietary changes, consider speaking to a therapist or counselor who specializes in gastrointestinal disorders.

3. **Support Groups:** Connecting with others who have IBS can provide a sense of community and understanding. Many online support groups and forums are

available where you can share experiences and coping strategies.

Conclusion: Finding Balance in Diet and Nutrition

As we conclude this chapter, remember that diet and nutrition are powerful tools in managing IBS. While the Low FODMAP diet and other dietary strategies can be effective, they should be undertaken with the guidance of a healthcare provider or dietitian.

Finding the right balance in your diet and nutrition can significantly improve your quality of life with IBS. It's about understanding your unique triggers, making informed food choices, and seeking support when needed.

In the chapters to come, we'll continue to explore various aspects of living with IBS, from the emotional impact to practical strategies for everyday life. Our goal is to provide you with the knowledge and tools you need to thrive, despite the challenges of IBS. So, stay with us as we continue our journey through the world of Irritable Bowel Syndrome.

CHAPTER 8

Living with IBS - Practical Tips and Emotional Well-Being

Welcome to the final chapter of our journey through the world of Irritable Bowel Syndrome (IBS). In this chapter, we'll explore practical tips for everyday life with IBS and delve into the emotional well-being aspects of living with this condition.

Practical Tips for Living with IBS

Living with IBS can present unique challenges, but there are practical strategies that can help you navigate everyday life more smoothly.

1. Bathroom Access: Plan your day to ensure easy access to a bathroom when needed. Knowing where restrooms are located in public places can reduce anxiety about finding one in a hurry.

2. Portable Essentials: Consider carrying a "IBS Kit" with essentials like toilet paper, wet wipes, and spare underwear in case of emergencies.

3. Food Preparation: Prepare meals at home whenever possible, as this allows you to control ingredients and portion sizes. It's also more comfortable to manage your dietary needs in a familiar environment.

4. Travel Considerations: When traveling, research bathroom locations in advance, and bring snacks or meals that align with your dietary restrictions. Inform your travel companions about your needs to avoid unnecessary stress.

5. Medication Management: If you take medications for IBS, ensure you have an adequate supply on hand, especially when traveling or during emergencies.

6. Stress Reduction: Incorporate stress-reduction techniques like mindfulness, deep breathing, or meditation into your daily routine to help manage the emotional impact of IBS.

7. Communication: Openly communicate with friends, family, and coworkers about your condition. Let them know how they can support you, such as understanding the need for bathroom breaks during outings.

8. Stay Informed: Keep yourself informed about IBS management strategies and treatment options. Knowledge empowers you to make informed decisions about your health.

Emotional Well-Being and IBS

The emotional aspect of living with IBS can't be overstated. The condition can affect your mental health, relationships, and overall well-being. Here's how to address the emotional side of IBS:

1. Seek Support: Don't hesitate to seek emotional support from friends, family, or a therapist who specializes in gastrointestinal disorders. Talking about your experiences can be cathartic and reduce feelings of isolation.

2. Mindfulness and Relaxation: Incorporate mindfulness and relaxation techniques into your daily routine to manage stress and anxiety. These practices can help you stay grounded and reduce the impact of emotional triggers on your symptoms.

3. Set Realistic Expectations: Understand that IBS can be unpredictable, and symptoms may fluctuate. Set realistic expectations for yourself and prioritize self-compassion.

4. Join Support Groups: Consider joining a local or online IBS support group where you can connect with others who understand your experiences. Sharing strategies and coping mechanisms can be invaluable.

5. Professional Help: If you're struggling with anxiety or depression related to IBS, consider seeking professional help. Therapists can provide coping strategies tailored to your specific emotional challenges.

6. Lifestyle Balance: Balance your lifestyle to include activities you enjoy and that promote emotional well-being. Engage in hobbies, spend time with loved ones, and practice self-care.

7. Keep a Symptom Diary: Maintaining a symptom diary can help you identify patterns and triggers, providing insights that can lead to better symptom management.

8. Manage Expectations: Understand that living with IBS may involve ups and downs. Managing expectations and focusing on improving your quality of life can reduce emotional distress.

Relationships and IBS

IBS can impact relationships with loved ones. Here's how to maintain healthy connections:

1. **Communication:** Openly communicate with your partner, friends, and family about your condition. Share your needs and preferences regarding diet, social activities, and emotional support.

2. **Education:** Provide your loved ones with educational resources about IBS to help them

understand the condition and its impact on your life.

3. Empathy: Encourage empathy and understanding in your relationships. Explain that IBS symptoms can be unpredictable and that you may need to make last-minute changes to plans.

4. Plan Together: When possible, involve your loved ones in planning meals and social activities that accommodate your dietary needs and IBS symptoms.

5. Seek Support Together: Encourage your loved ones to join support groups or attend therapy sessions with you if they're interested. This can help them gain insights into your experiences and offer better support.

Employment and IBS

Managing IBS in the workplace can be challenging, but there are strategies to help:

1. **Open Communication:** Communicate with your employer or supervisor about your condition. Discuss any accommodations you may need, such as access to a restroom or flexible work hours.

2. Bathroom Access: Make sure you're aware of the nearest restroom locations in your workplace. This can help reduce anxiety about bathroom emergencies.

3. Stress Reduction at Work: Incorporate stress-reduction techniques into your workday, such as deep breathing exercises or brief mindfulness breaks.

4. Dietary Considerations: Plan your meals and snacks to align with your dietary needs while at work. Avoid foods that trigger your symptoms.

5. Remote Work: If possible, consider remote work options that provide more flexibility and a comfortable environment.

Life Beyond IBS

While IBS can be a significant part of your life, it doesn't define you. Remember that you are not your condition. Embrace activities, passions, and relationships that bring joy and fulfillment into your life.

CONCLUSION

Thriving Despite IBS

As we conclude our journey through the world of Irritable Bowel Syndrome, remember that living with IBS is about more than just managing symptoms. It's about finding balance in your diet, nurturing your emotional well-being, and maintaining meaningful relationships.

By incorporating practical tips, seeking support, and focusing on your overall quality of life, you can thrive despite the challenges of IBS. Your journey is unique, and you have the strength to navigate it successfully.

Thank you for joining us on this exploration of IBS. We hope this guide has provided you with valuable insights and tools to enhance your journey towards a healthier, more fulfilling life with IBS.

In concluding our journey through the pages of this book on Irritable Bowel Syndrome (IBS), we arrive at a pivotal point in our understanding of this complex condition. We've explored IBS from its roots, understanding its intricacies, its various subtypes, and the many facets of managing life with IBS.

IBS is not merely a gastrointestinal ailment; it's a condition that intertwines physical symptoms with emotional challenges. It's a reminder that our bodies and minds are profoundly interconnected.

We've learned about the importance of personalized approaches to diagnosis, treatment, and management. No two individuals experience IBS in exactly the same way, and there is no one-size-fits-all solution. Instead, we've emphasized the significance of tailored strategies, whether in diet, stress management, or medication, guided by healthcare professionals who understand the nuances of the condition.

Through our exploration of diet and nutrition, we've witnessed the transformative power of food choices. The Low FODMAP diet, in particular, has emerged as a promising tool, showcasing how understanding your body's unique responses to certain foods can lead to improved symptom management. We've also highlighted the role of mindfulness, relaxation, and emotional support in the journey towards better living with IBS.

The emotional aspect of IBS cannot be overstated. Living with a condition that affects one's daily life, social interactions, and even mental health requires resilience, empathy, and understanding. We've stressed the importance of seeking support, whether from friends, family, or mental health professionals, to navigate the emotional challenges that IBS presents.

In relationships and the workplace, we've seen the

significance of open communication and empathy. IBS can impact not only individuals but also those around them. By fostering understanding and involving loved ones in your journey, you can build stronger, more supportive connections.

Finally, we've explored the practical aspects of managing IBS in everyday life, from bathroom access to travel considerations. These are the real-life strategies that can make a tangible difference in the quality of life for individuals with IBS.

As we conclude this book, let us remember that IBS is a part of life, but it is not life itself. It does not define you. You are not your condition. With the knowledge and tools provided in these pages, you have the strength to thrive, to embrace the activities, passions, and relationships that bring joy and fulfillment into your life.

May this book serve as a beacon of understanding and empowerment, guiding you on your journey towards a healthier, more vibrant life with IBS. Your journey is unique, but you are not alone. Together, let us face the challenges of IBS with courage, resilience, and hope.